17 Day Diet Recipes

50 Delicious Recipes for the 17 Day Diet Plan
+ Our Free 17 Day Diet Summary

Get the Secret 17 Day Diet Recipes that Everyone is
Looking for:

M. Smith & R. King
Edited by: Country Cooking Publishing

17 Day Diet Recipes - 50 Delicious Recipes for the 17 Day Diet Plan + Our Free 17 Day Diet Summary

Copyright © 2011 by M. Smith & R. King

Table of Contents

17 Day Diet Summary 1

Strawberry Kefir Shake 8

Scrumptious Pie Smoothie 10

Berry Smoothie 12

Very Berry Shake 14

Breakfast Omelet 16

Apple Breakfast Cakes 18

Spinach Breakfast Pizza 20

Veggie Scramble..22

Spicy Turkey Burgers 24

Chicken and Fruit Wraps..26

Tuna Slaw..28

Green Bean Salad..30

Everything Salad 32

Spinach and Egg Salad 34

Simple Vegetable Salad 36

Mexican Salad...38

Baked Chicken Soup 40

Turkey Chili Soup...42

Three Veggie Lunch Cups...44

Baked Eggplant...46

Grilled Herbed Turkey Breasts...48

Turkey Vegetable Hodgepodge 50

Asparagus Stuffed Turkey 52

Baked Turkey and Tomato Peppers 54

Stuffed Chicken 56

Seasoned Chicken & Vegetables 58

Mushroom Chicken...60

Herbed Tilapia 62

Baked Salmon..64

Broiled Flounder..66

Stir Fry Shrimp Veggies..68

Cherry Tomato Scampi..70

Slow Cooked Shredded Pork 72

Taco Meatballs 74

Sweet Potato Wedges...76

Smoked Paprika Cabbage 78

Mushroom Green Beans 80

Sautéed Eggplant Fries 82

Spiced Cauliflower...84

Lemon Artichokes 86

Cinnamon Pudding 88

Pumpkin Dessert 90

Raspberry Tea Gelatin Bites.......................................92

Nutmeg Drops 94

Crispy Snack Chips...96

Applesauce Cookies..98

Vegetable Dip... 100

Spinach Muffins 102

Homemade Spice.. 104

Quick Homemade Salsa... 106

CopyCat Restaurant Recipes 108

17 Day Diet Summary

If you are looking for a way to lose weight quickly and efficiently the 17 Day Diet may be just what you need. Introduced by Dr. Michael Moreno, aka "Dr. Mike", as a jump start diet, it allows you to quickly lose weight but also gives you mental boost most other diets don't. It can be difficult to feel the mental side of a diet. Many diets take months to start showing their true effects but this diet helps you in a matter of days.

The diet includes eating fruits, vegetables and lean meats. It cuts out foods that are full of sugars, fats and overly salty foods. Sounds boring huh? That's the beauty of this diet; it only takes 17 days meaning there's not much chance of it becoming boring or stagnate. With just a little over 2 weeks this diet can keep you from slipping back into your old ways and shows results fast.

You also won't feel those dreaded hunger pains that many diets leave you with. By eating the right foods you have a full stomach and not feel those anguished pains that many diets leave you with. It helps to boost energy levels as well. There are normally no plateaus with this diet as you find with many other diets today. Because you vary the foods you eat and in turn the calories you ingest the body can't adapt and become stuck. This keeps your body from becoming bored so the weight melts away at a rapid pace.

So what's behind this diet that makes it so successful? It's simple. 3 cycles of 17 days each and a fourth cycle that is ongoing to help you keep the weight off. Cycle 1 is the Accelerate cycle. This cycle helps to remove sugars and fats from the body.

Cycle 1 cleanses the body removing not only fats and sugars but toxins as well. It limits the amount of carbohydrates ingested by removing white bread, rice, potatoes and pasta. No chocolate or other sweet desserts are allowed. This insures that your body can metabolize the fat stored and helps your body to tap into its own supply of fat.

Cycle 1 allows you to enjoy foods that are a high source of protein. Fish, eggs, poultry and vegetables such as bell peppers, broccoli, cabbage, onions, tomatoes and spinach are just a few. These types of vegetables help clean the blood, liver and intestines of toxins and unwanted fatty cells.

Two servings of low sugar fruits such as apples, pears, red grapes and all types of berries are allowed in Cycle 1. These fruits are low in calories but full of fiber and water. Plain yogurt, low fat acidophilus milk, cottage cheese and low sodium miso as well as low sodium broth are also allowed to help clean the digestive system.

Cycle 2 is the Activate cycle. This cycle helps to rest the body metabolism so that it retains the fat burning process. Many diets allow your body to begin changing but because the body can adapt so easily the weight loss begins to plateau. This cycle prevents that from happening.

On this cycle you may continue to eat all the foods you enjoyed on the Accelerate cycle while adding a few more delightful treats. Foods such as shellfish and lean cuts of beef, pork and lamb can be enjoyed in this cycle. Brown rice, bulgur and pearled barley are also added. Old fashioned oatmeal, grits and cream of wheat are also allowed in this cycle.

All kinds of beans and peas as well as corn, sweet potatoes and squashes are also a part of this cycle. Low sodium broths, lite soy sauce, low car ketchup and fat free sour cream may also be used in moderation. Natural carbs are also a part of this cycle and spices are allowed giving your body something that's not only healthy but tastes great also.

Cycle 3 or the Achieve cycle teaches you to control your portions while adding a fitness regime to the diet. New foods are added and the rules are fewer but it helps you to achieve better eating habits. Habits such as including healthy foods, eating at regular times and watching the amount you eat are a big part of this cycle.

With cycles 1 and 2 you will see a fast drop in weight but in cycle 3 your weight loss will begin to slow down. That's okay because the weight you have lost over the 34 days of cycle 1 and 2 should have you very close to your desired weight. Cycle 3 will help you lose a little more but will also help you start the process of maintaining your desired weight.

The Achieve Cycle lets you add foods such as pasta, whole grain breads, fruits and snacks. You may also enjoy one alcoholic drink a day if you like. Just remember that alcohol can dehydrate and can cause water weight that will up your daily weight on the scales. So if you want to maintain your weight or continue to lose alcohol may not be the best for your particular needs.

Again this cycle lasts for 17 days. More types of foods are allowed so portion control is very important. Keep meat portions small, remove the skin from poultry, eat as many egg whites as you like but try to keep the yolks down to four a week. Enjoy fresh fruits, frozen fruits and canned fruits. Any frozen or canned fruits should be unsweetened.

You don't have to eat all the foods allowed in one day. Stretch them out so you can have an enjoyable meal every day. Eating slowly and enjoying your foods is something to savor on this cycle. You want to be full but not overly stuffed. Also increase your exercise to 30 minutes sessions.

Cycle 4 is the Arrive Cycle where you can congratulate yourself for a job well done. Sticking to the 17 Day Diet for the first 3 cycles have brought you results but now you need to maintain those results for the rest of your life. On this cycle you can eat from your favorite foods on the weekends and still maintain the body you have worked so hard to achieve.

Foods that are included in Cycles 1, 2 and 3 are allows on weekdays. On the weekends you can enjoy any of your favorite foods in moderation. Broth based soups, unsweetened fruit juices and vegetable juices are also allowed. Panning is an important part of this cycle to keep those spur-of-the-moment urges to a minimum.

The 17 Day Diet is not only quick but it's very simple. Sticking to the 3 cycles for 17 days each can bring fast results as well as a healthier eating lifestyle. You goals can be achieved and your life can be happier and healthier by eating the right foods in the right amounts. If you're look for a diet that stands out in weight loss, mind building and a healthier lifestyle this diet may be just what the doctor ordered.

17 Day Diet Recipes

Strawberry Kefir Shake

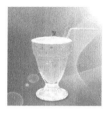

Ingredients:

4 ice cubes

Water

1 C strawberry kefir

2 packets of Truvia sweetener

Strawberry Kefir Shake

Directions:

Place the ice cubes into a 2 cup measuring cup.

Add enough water to bring the level to the 2 cup mark.

Pour the water/ice into the blender.

Add the kefir and Truvia to the blender.

Blend on high until creamy.

Pour into a milk shake glass and enjoy.

Scrumptious Pie Smoothie

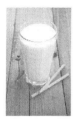

Ingredients:

1 (6 oz.) container of plain yogurt

1 small apple, peeled and diced

¼ tsp. pumpkin pie spice

¼ tsp. apple pie spice

1 dash of vanilla

1 packet of Truvia sweetener

Directions:

Place the yogurt and apple into the blender.

Sprinkle in both spices.

Add the vanilla and Truvia.

Blend until very smooth

Berry Smoothie

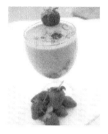

Ingredients:

1 C of unsweetened kefir

1 C frozen unsweetened mixed berries

1 tbsp. sugar free strawberry jam

Berry Smoothie

Directions:

Place the kefir into the blender.

Add the berries and jam.

Blend until smooth.

Very Berry Shake

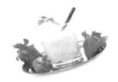

Ingredients:

1 (6 oz.) container of sugar free fruit flavored yogurt

1 C acidophilus milk

2 C frozen berries, unsweetened

Very Berry Shake

Directions:

Place the yogurt into the blender.

Add the milk and berries.

Blend until smooth.

Breakfast Omelet

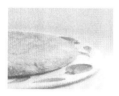

Ingredients:

2 eggs

1 tbsp. water

1 tsp. vanilla

2 packets Truvia sweetener

1 tsp. cinnamon

Directions:

Break the eggs into a bowl and whisk in the water and vanilla.

Heat a skillet over medium heat.

Add the eggs and cook for 3 minutes or until set.

Flip the eggs and cook an additional 2 minutes until completely set and fluffy.

Remove the eggs to a serving plate.

Stir together the Truvia and cinnamon until well blended.

Sprinkle the mixture over the hot omelet.

Apple Breakfast Cakes

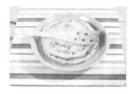

Ingredients:

1 egg

2 egg whites

¼ tsp. cinnamon

1/8 tsp. nutmeg

1 small apple, peeled and chopped fine

Directions:

Break the egg into a bowl and lightly.

Add the egg whites and whisk until blended in well.

Whisk in the cinnamon and nutmeg.

Add the apples and stir to combine.

Heat a non-stick skillet over medium heat.

Pour 1/3 of the egg mixture into the heated pan.

Cook the mixture for 5 minutes or until set.

Flip and cook until lightly browned.

Continue with the remaining egg mixture until all the mixture has been used.

Spinach Breakfast Pizza

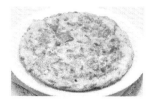

Ingredients:

2 egg whites

1/8 tsp. salt

1/8 tsp. pepper

¼ C fresh spinach, chopped

1/8 C tomato, chopped

Directions:

Place the egg whites into a bowl and sprinkle with the salt and pepper.

Beat the egg whites with a whisk until just frothy.

Stir in the spinach and tomato.

Heat a skillet over medium heat.

Pour the egg mixture into the skillet and cook 5 minutes or until the eggs are cooked through.

Remove to a plate with a spatula and enjoy.

Veggie Scramble

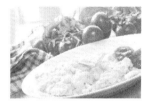

Ingredients:

4 egg whites, lightly beaten

1/8 tsp. salt

1/8 tsp. pepper

1/8 C red onion, chopped fine

1/8 C tomatoes, diced fine

1 tbsp. low fat feta cheese, shredded

Veggie Scramble

Directions:

Season the lightly beaten eggs with the salt and pepper.

Add the onions and tomatoes and stir to combine.

Stir in the cheese.

Heat a non-stick skillet over medium low heat.

Add the eggs and cook 2 minutes or until beginning to set.

With a fork scramble the eggs and continue cooking 2 minutes or until the eggs are cooked through.

Spicy Turkey Burgers

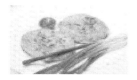

Ingredients:

1 tbsp. hot sauce

2 tsp. cumin, ground

2 tsp. chili powder

1 garlic clove, minced

1/8 tsp. salt

1 lb. ground turkey

Spicy Turkey Burgers

Directions:

In a bowl whisk together the hot sauce, cumin, chili powder, garlic and salt until well blended.

Crumble the turkey into the mixture and using your hands work the hot sauce mixture into the turkey well.

Form the mixture into patties.

Heat a non-stick skillet over medium heat.

Add the patties and cook 5 minutes.

Flip the patties and continue to cook for 4 minutes or until the patties are cooked through.

Chicken and Fruit Wraps

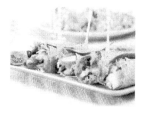

Ingredients:

1 chicken breast, cooked and cut into pieces

1 scallion, diced

2 tbsp. celery, chopped

1 tbsp. olive oil

1/8 tsp. salt

1/8 tsp. pepper

4 fresh lettuce leaves

½ C of fresh peach slices

Directions:

Place the chicken into a bowl.

Add the scallion, celery, oil, salt and pepper and stir to combine well.

Refrigerate 1 hour until well chilled.

Place the lettuce leaves onto a serving plate.

Spoon the chicken mixture down the middle of each leaf.

Add the peaches to the top.

Wrap the lettuce around the filling and secure with a toothpick.

Tuna Slaw

Ingredients:

¾ C cabbage, shredded

¼ C carrots, shredded

1 (5 oz.) can of tuna in water, drained well

2 tbsp. plain yogurt

2 tsp. fat free ranch dressing

Directions:

Place the cabbage and carrots into a serving bowl and toss to combine.

Gently fold in the tuna.

In a separate bowl mix together the yogurt and ranch dressing.

Stir the yogurt mixture into the cabbage/tuna mixture until well coated.

Refrigerate for at least 1 hour or until chilled through.

Green Bean Salad

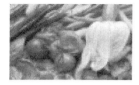

Ingredients:

2 C of fresh lettuce, torn

1 C of cooked green beans

1 small tomato, chopped

1 small cucumber, sliced

2 scallions, chopped

1 tbsp. olive oil

2 tbsp. balsamic vinegar

Directions:

Place the lettuce into a bowl.

Add the green beans, tomato, cucumber and scallion and toss gently to combine.

Whisk together the oil and vinegar in a small bowl.

Drizzle the mixture evenly over the salad and toss to coat.

Everything Salad

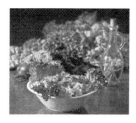

Ingredients:

3 C of lettuce, all varieties torn

1 large cucumber, sliced

1 large tomato, wedged

1 large onion, sliced thin

1 small head of cauliflower, broken into small pieces

2 carrots, sliced thin

1 stalk of celery, sliced thin

¼ C watercress

2 hard-boiled eggs, chopped

1 (6 oz.) can of light tuna in water, drained well

4 tbsp. flaxseed oil

8 tbsp. balsamic vinegar

Directions:

Place the lettuce into a large salad bowl.

Add the remaining vegetables and toss to combine.

Add the tuna and toss to combine into the salad well.

Whisk together the flaxseed oil and vinegar.

Drizzle the dressing over the top and toss to coat.

Spinach and Egg Salad

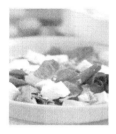

Ingredients:

2 C baby spinach leaves, torn

2 hard-boiled eggs, sliced

2 tbsp. reduced fat feta cheese

1 tbsp. olive oil

2 tbsp. balsamic vinegar

Directions:

Place the spinach into a bowl.

Add the eggs and cheese and toss to combine.

Whisk together the oil and vinegar well.

Pour the dressing over the salad and toss again to coat well.

Simple Vegetable Salad

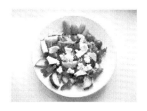

Ingredients:

2 tomatoes, chopped

½ tsp. salt

1 pk. fresh baby carrots

1 cucumber, sliced

1 small red onion, chopped

½ tsp. oregano

1 tbsp. olive oil

2 tbsp. low fat feta cheese, crumbled

Directions:

Place the tomatoes into a bowl and sprinkle evenly with the salt.

Allow the tomatoes to sit for 2 minutes.

Add the carrots, cucumber and red onions to the tomatoes and toss.

Sprinkle with the oregano and toss again.

Pour the oil over the top and toss gently to coat.

Spread the feta cheese over the salad just before serving.

Mexican Salad

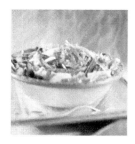

Ingredients:

1 lb. lean ground turkey

1 envelope of taco seasoning

1 C lettuce, torn

1 C tomatoes, chopped

1 C red onion, chopped

¼ C reduce fat cheddar cheese, shredded

Directions:

Crumble the turkey into a skillet placed over medium heat.

Stirring often, brown the turkey for 6 minutes or until completely cooked through.

Sprinkle the seasoning mix over the turkey and stir to coat well.

Place the lettuce into a bowl.

Spoon the meat over the lettuce.

Add the tomatoes, onions and cheese.

Baked Chicken Soup

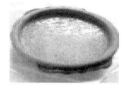

Ingredients:

1 C of cabbage, torn into bite size pieces

1 C okra, sliced

1 onion, chopped

2 celery stalks, chopped

1 (14 oz.) can fat free chicken broth

1 tsp. salt

½ tsp. pepper

3 chicken breasts, baked and cut into pieces

Directions:

Place the cabbage, okra, onion and celery into a soup pot.

Pour in the broth and sprinkle with the salt and pepper.

Place the pan over medium heat and simmer for 30 minutes or until the vegetables are tender.

Add the chicken and simmer an additional 15 minutes or until the chicken is heated through.

Turkey Chili Soup

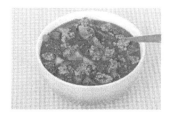

Ingredients:

1 lb. ground turkey

1 C onion, chopped

1 C green bell pepper, chopped

1 C tomatoes, diced

2 C tomato sauce

1 tbsp. chili powder

½ tsp. salt

Directions:

Crumble the ground turkey into a large saucepan placed over medium high heat.

Cook, stirring often, for 6 minutes or until the turkey is browned through.

Add the onion, bell pepper and tomatoes.

Stir in the tomato sauce.

Sprinkle in the chili powder and salt and stir to combine.

Simmer over low heat for 30 minutes, stirring occasionally, or until heated through.

2 C of beans may be added in with the vegetables for Cycle 2 and 3.

Three Veggie Lunch Cups

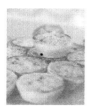

Ingredients:

1 (10 oz.) pkg. frozen spinach

2 eggs, lightly beaten

¼ C green bell pepper, chopped

2 tbsp. onion, chopped

½ C low fat Parmesan cheese, grated

Three Veggie Lunch Cups

Directions:

Preheat the oven to 350 degrees and line a 6 cup muffin tin with paper liners.

Place the spinach into a microwave safe bowl and microwave on high for 2 minutes.

Remove the spinach and let cool just enough to handle.

Squeeze out any excess moisture from the spinach and chop.

Place the spinach, green peppers and onions into a bowl.

Add the egg and cheese and stir until blended together well.

Fill each paper lined muffin cup 2/3 full of the mixture.

Bake 20 minutes or until a butter knife inserted in the center comes out clean.

Let cool slightly and serve immediately.

Baked Eggplant

Ingredients:

2 eggplants, peeled and cut in half

6 egg whites

4 tbsp. water

1 C fat free Parmesan cheese, grated

1 tsp. garlic powder

2 C low carb marinara sauce

Directions:

Preheat the oven to 400 degrees and spray a 13X9 baking dish with a non-stick cooking spray.

Place the egg whites into a dish.

Add the water and whisk until frothy.

Place the Parmesan cheese into a large bowl.

Dip the eggplant into the egg mixture and allow any excess to drip off.

Roll the eggplant through the cheese until completely covered.

Place the eggplant into the prepared baking dish.

Sprinkle the garlic powder evenly over the eggplant.

Bake 30 minutes, turning once, or until the eggplant is tender and lightly browned.

Pour the marinara sauce over the top of the eggplant and bake 20 minutes or until the sauce is bubbly.

Grilled Herbed Turkey Breasts

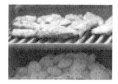

Ingredients:

3 garlic cloves, minced

2 tbsp. olive oil

2 tbsp. lemon juice

1 tsp. rosemary, crushed

1 tsp. thyme, crushed

1 tsp. oregano, crushed

1 lb. turkey breast, sliced

Directions:

In a small bowl stir together the olive oil and lemon juice.

Add the rosemary, thyme and oregano and stir to blend in well.

Brush the mixture over both sides of turkey slices and let stand 20 minutes.

Heat the grill to medium low heat.

Place the turkey slices onto the hot grill and grill for 2 minutes.

Flip the turkey slices over and continue to grill 2 minutes or until cooked through.

Turkey Vegetable Hodgepodge

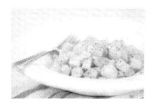

Ingredients:

1 tbsp. olive oil

1 lb. turkey breast, cubed

1 green pepper, diced

1 carrot, cubed small

1 C of cabbage, chopped

1small onion, chopped

1 stalk of celery, chopped

1 tsp. garlic powder,

1 tsp. allspice

½ tsp. cumin

¼ tsp. cayenne pepper

1 C fat free chicken broth

Directions:

Pour the oil into a skillet over medium heat.

Add the turkey cubes, stirring often cook 8 minutes or until lightly browned and cooked through.

Add the vegetables and spices and stir well.

Cook the mixture, stirring almost constantly, for 5 minutes or until hot.

Pour in the chicken broth and stir to mix all the ingredients together well.

Cover and simmer over low heat for 10 minutes.

Asparagus Stuffed Turkey

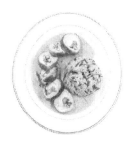

Ingredients:

1 (3 lb.) frozen turkey breast, thawed

8 asparagus spears, steamed and cut into 4 pieces each

8 baby carrots, cut into strips and steamed

6 scallions, chopped

¼ tsp. salt

½ tsp. pepper

¼ C low sodium, fat free chicken broth

Directions:

Preset the oven temperature to 350 degrees and preheat the oven.

Cut the turkey into 8 pieces.

Lay the turkey pieces out on parchment paper and pound to about a 1 inch thickness.

In a bowl toss together the asparagus, carrots and scallions.

Sprinkle with the salt and pepper and stir to mix in well.

Spread the mixture over each piece of the turkey breast leaving a 1 inch area of meat uncovered at the bottom.

Starting at the top of each piece, roll the turkey around the asparagus mixture tightly.

Place seam side down into a baking dish Pour the chicken broth over the top and cover the pan tightly with foil.

Bake 25 minutes or until the turkey has cooked through.

Remove the foil and bake an additional 3 minutes or starting to brown slightly.

Baked Turkey and Tomato Peppers

Ingredients:

4 bell peppers

1 lb. ground turkey

1 onion, chopped

1 garlic clove, minced

4 small tomatoes, chopped

1 egg white, lightly beaten

¼ tsp. salt

¼ tsp. pepper

1/8 tsp. red pepper flakes

Baked Turkey and Tomato Peppers

Directions:

Preset the oven to 350 degrees.

Wash the peppers, cut out the tops and remove the seeds and membranes.

Parboil the peppers in a pan of boiling salted water for 3 minutes.

Remove the peppers and drain well.

Crumble the turkey into a mixing bowl.

Add the onion, garlic, tomatoes, egg, salt, pepper and red pepper and mix well.

Stuff each pepper with ¼ of the mixture.

Stand the pepper cut side up in a baking dish and cover with foil.

Bake the peppers for 20 minutes.

Remove the foil and continue baking 15 minutes or until the turkey is cooked through.

Stuffed Chicken

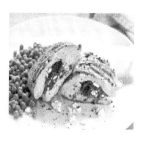

Ingredients:

2 boneless, skinless chicken breasts

1 tsp. garlic powder

1 tbsp. olive oil

1 (10 oz.) pkg. spinach, thawed and squeezed dry

1 small onion, chopped

2 tbsp. fat free feta cheese, crumbled

1 C Greek yogurt

Stuffed Chicken

Directions:

Set the oven to 350 degrees and preheat.

Pound the chicken breasts out so they are very thin.

Sprinkle both sides of each piece of chicken with the garlic powder.

Place the olive oil in a skillet and heat until hot.

Add the spinach and onions and sauté for 3 minutes until the spinach is wilted.

Remove from the skillet and cool slightly.

Add the yogurt to the spinach mixture and stir well.

Sprinkle both chicken breasts with the crumbled cheese.

Roll the chicken around the filling and secure with a tooth-pick.

Place the rolled chicken in a baking dish and cover tightly with foil.

Bake 30 minutes or until the chicken is cooked through.

Seasoned Chicken & Vegetables

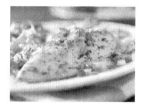

Ingredients:

1 C carrots, chopped

1 C onions, chopped

½ C celery, chopped

½ C low sodium, low fat chicken broth

1 tsp. Italian seasoning

2 lbs. boneless, skinless chicken breasts

½ tsp. salt

½ tsp. pepper

1 (14.5 oz.) can no salt petite diced tomatoes

Directions:

Place the carrots, onions and celery into a slow cooker.

Pour the broth over the top.

Sprinkle in the Italian seasoning.

Season the chicken on all sides with the salt and pepper.

Lay the seasoned chicken over the top of the vegetables.

Pour the tomatoes, with their juice, over the top of the chicken.

Cover the slow cooker and cook on low for 8 hours or until the chicken has cooked through.

Mushroom Chicken

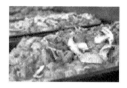

Ingredients:

1 tsp. olive oil

1 tsp. lemon juice

1 garlic clove, minced

¼ tsp. pepper

2 boneless skinless chicken breasts

1tsp water

½ C of onion, diced

1 C of mushrooms, sliced

Directions:

Place the oil, lemon juice, garlic and pepper into a bowl and whisk to combine.

Put the chicken breasts into a skillet placed over medium heat.

Pour the oil mixture over the top of the chicken.

Cook the chicken for 6 minutes.

Turn the chicken and cook for an additional 5 minutes or until the chicken is cooked through.

Remove the chicken to a plate.

Add the water to the skillet and stir to loosen any brown bits in the skillet.

Add the onions and mushrooms and cook, stirring often, for 5 minutes or until tender.

Add the chicken back to the skillet and cook on low until heated through.

Herbed Tilapia

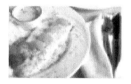

Ingredients:

1 tbsp. olive oil

Juice from lemon

2 tsp. oregano

½ tsp. paprika

¼ tsp. salt

¼ tsp. pepper

4 fresh tilapia fillets

Herbed Tilapia

Directions:

Set the oven to 400 degrees and preheat.

Pour the oil into a bowl.

Add the lemon juice, oregano, paprika, salt and pepper.

Place the tilapia fillets in a single layer in a baking dish.

Pour the oil mixture over the top.

Cover the dish tightly with foil.

Bake the fillets for 15 minutes or until cooked through.

Baked Salmon

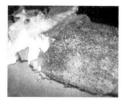

Ingredients:

2 salmon fillets

1 tbsp. olive oil

2 garlic cloves, chopped

½ C lemon juice

1 tsp. oregano

Baked Salmon

Directions:

Preheat the oven to 350 degrees and spay a baking dish with cooking spray.

Place the salmon into the prepared baking dish.

Pour the oil over the top of the salmon fillets.

Spread the chopped garlic over the top of each of the fillets.

Pour in the lemon juice and sprinkle with oregano.

Bake 25 minutes or until the salmon is cooked through.

Broiled Flounder

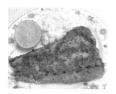

Ingredients:

2 tbsp. olive oil

2 tbsp. rice wine vinegar

2 tbsp. lite soy sauce

1 tsp. garlic, minced

1 lb. flounder fillets

2 tbsp. sesame seeds

Directions:

Preheat the broiler and spray a broiler pan well with a non-stick cooking spray.

Whisk together the oil, vinegar, soy sauce and garlic in a large bowl.

Dip the fillets into the mixture being sure they are coated well.

Place the fillets onto the prepared broiler pan.

Sprinkle the sesame seeds evenly over the fish.

Broil the fish on the lowest oven rack for 15 minutes, turning once, or until the fish is cooked through and flakes easily with a fork.

Stir Fry Shrimp Veggies

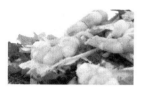

Ingredients:

1 lb. fresh large shrimp peeled and deveined

3 tbsp. red wine vinegar

3 tbsp. low sodium soy sauce

3 tbsp. water

1 tbsp. cornstarch

1 packet of Truvia sweetener

1 tbsp. olive oil

2 garlic cloves, minced

2 C broccoli florets

1 C carrot, shredded

1 small onion, sliced thin

1 C mushrooms, sliced

Stir Fry Shrimp Veggies

Directions:

Rinse shrimp and pat dry.

In a bowl combine the vinegar, soy sauce, water, cornstarch and Truvia.

Place the oil in a skillet and heat to hot but not smoking.

Stir in the garlic and cook 15 seconds or until fragrant.

Stir in the broccoli, carrot and onions and cook 3 minutes stirring almost constantly.

Add the mushrooms and stir fry for 1 minute or until the veggies are crisp tender.

Remove the vegetables and add the vinegar mixture.

Bring the mixture to a boil then add the shrimp.

Cook the shrimp, stirring constantly, for 3 minutes or until the shrimp turn opaque.

Return the vegetables and cook 2 minutes or until heated through.

Cherry Tomato Scampi

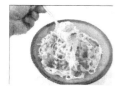

Ingredients:

2 tsp. olive oil

¾ lb. shrimp, peeled and deveined

½ tsp. salt

1 tbsp. parsley, chopped

1 garlic clove, minced

8 cherry tomatoes, halved

¼ C low sodium chicken broth

2 tbsp. lemon juice

1 tbsp. low fat Parmesan cheese, grated

Cherry Tomato Scampi

Directions:

Heat the oil in a skillet over medium high heat.

Add the shrimp and sprinkle evenly with the salt.

Cook the shrimp, stirring often for 5 minutes or until pink and cooked through.

Remove the shrimp and set aside.

Reduce the heat to medium and stir in the parsley and garlic.

Cook the mixture, stirring often, for 1 minute or until the garlic is fragrant.

Stir in the tomatoes, chicken broth and lemon juice.

Cover the pan and cook 3 minutes or until the tomatoes are soft.

Return the shrimp to the pan and cook uncovered until heated through.

Sprinkle with the Parmesan just before serving and serve over whole wheat noodles.

Slow Cooked Shredded Pork

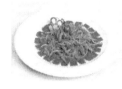

Ingredients:

1 (4 lb.) center cut boneless pork loin roast

1 ½ tsp. salt, divided

½ tsp. pepper

1 C of water

1 ½ C cider vinegar

½ C low fat ketchup

2 packets of Truvia sweetener

½ tsp. cayenne pepper

Slow Cooked Shredded Pork

Directions:

Sprinkle the roast on all sides with ½ tsp. salt and the pepper.

Place the roast in the crock pot and add the water.

Cover and cook on low for 9 hours or until cooked through.

Remove the roast and allow it to cool just enough to handle, then shred.

Return the shredded pork to the crock pot.

In a bowl mix together the vinegar and ketchup.

Add the Truvia and cayenne pepper and stir to blend in well.

Pour just enough of the sauce over the meat to coat well.

Cover and adjust the heat to high on the crock pot.

Cook 30 minutes or until heated through.

Serve with the remaining sauce on the side.

Taco Meatballs

Ingredients:

1 lb. extra lean ground beef

1 packet taco seasoning mix

1 tbsp. olive oil

2 C of low fat salsa

Directions:

Crumble the meat into a mixing bowl.

Sprinkle the taco seasoning over the meat and mix well to combine.

Form the meat mixture into balls.

Pour the olive oil into a skillet and heat over medium high heat.

Add the meatballs and stirring occasionally, cook for 10 minutes or until cooked through.

Remove the meatballs to paper towel to drain.

Return the meatballs to the skillet and pour the salsa over the top.

Heat the meatballs and sauce for 5 minutes or until heated through.

Sweet Potato Wedges

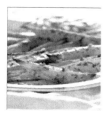

Ingredients:

4 sweet potatoes cut into wedges

½ tsp. salt

½ cumin

¼ tsp. cayenne pepper

1 tbsp. olive oil

Directions:

Place the sweet potatoes into a bowl of cold water and let stand 30 minutes.

Set the oven to 400 degrees and preheat.

Remove the sweet potato wedges and pat dry with paper towel.

Place the wedges into a bowl.

Sprinkle evenly with the salt, cumin and cayenne pepper.

Drizzle with the olive oil and toss to coat well.

Spread the wedges in a single layer onto an ungreased baking sheet.

Bake 20 minutes, turning often for even crisping.

Smoked Paprika Cabbage

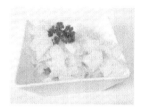

Ingredients:

1 head of cabbage, cut into small pieces

1 small onion, sliced

½ C of water

1 tsp. smoked paprika

2 tbsp. olive oil

Directions:

Place the cabbage into a large pot.

Add the water and place the pot over high heat.

Bring the water to a boil and boil until the water is almost gone and the cabbage is tender.

Reduce the heat to low.

Sprinkle the paprika evenly over the cabbage.

Add the oil and stir to coat the cabbage well.

Stir and cook 2 minutes or until heated through.

Mushroom Green Beans

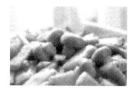

Ingredients:

1 (16 oz.) pkg. frozen green beans

1 tsp. olive oil

1 white onion, diced

1 (6 oz.) pkg. button mushrooms

½ tsp. pepper

Mushroom Green Beans

Directions:

Microwave the green beans as directed on the package.

Place the oil into a skillet over medium heat.

Add the onion and mushrooms.

Cook the vegetables, stirring often, for 5 minutes or until the onions start to caramelize.

Stir in the green beans and cook 1 minute or until heated through.

Sprinkle with the pepper and stir.

Sautéed Eggplant Fries

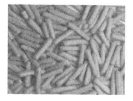

Ingredients:

1 tbsp. olive oil

2 eggs, lightly beaten

½ tsp. salt

1 small eggplant, cut into fries

Directions:

Place the oil in a skillet over medium high heat.

Sprinkle the salt into the beaten egg and whisk to combine.

Dip the eggplant fries into the egg mixture and allow any excess to drain off.

Sauté the eggplant pieces in the hot oil, turning often, for 4 minutes or until nice and crispy.

Spiced Cauliflower

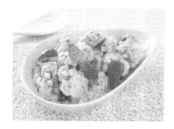

Ingredients:

1 head of cauliflower

1 tbsp. olive oil

2 tsp. cumin seeds

2 tsp. turmeric, ground

1 red onion, chopped

2 garlic cloves, chopped

1 tsp. parsley, chopped

¼ tsp. pepper

Mint leaves

Spiced Cauliflower

Directions:

Clean the cauliflower and break into small pieces.

Place the oil in a skillet over medium heat.

Stir in the cumin seeds and turmeric and cook stirring often for 3 minutes or until the cumin seeds begin to pop.

Stir in the onion and garlic and cook 3 minutes or until the onion is just beginning to tender.

Add the cauliflower, reduce the heat to medium low and cover the skillet.

Cook 5 minutes or until the cauliflower is fork tender.

Sprinkle with the pepper and stir to combine.

Garnish with the mint leaves just before serving.

Lemon Artichokes

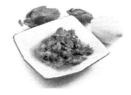

Ingredients:

4 artichokes

¼ C of lemon juice

Directions:

Place the artichokes into a large saucepan.

Add just enough water to cover the artichokes.

Pour the lemon juice into the water.

Place the pan over high heat and bring to a boil.

Reduce the heat to low, cover the pan and cook 1 hour or until the artichokes are tender.

Drain well and let cool slightly before serving.

Cinnamon Pudding

Ingredients:

1 C low fat Greek yogurt

1 tsp. vanilla

2 packets of Truvia

1 tsp. cinnamon

Cinnamon Pudding

Directions:

Place the yogurt into a bowl.

Add the vanilla and Truvia and stir until blended in well.

Sprinkle the cinnamon over the top.

Pumpkin Dessert

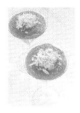

Ingredients:

1 (6 oz.) container of plain yogurt

1 packet of Truvia sweetener

¼ tsp. pumpkin pie spice

Pumpkin Dessert

Directions:

Spoon the yogurt in a bowl.

Sprinkle the Truvia and pumpkin spice over the yogurt and stir to combine.

Raspberry Tea Gelatin Bites

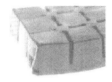

Ingredients:

1 envelope Know unflavored gelatin

1 C boiling water

1 sleeve Crystal Light raspberry green tea mix

1 C of cold water

Directions:

Stir the unflavored gelatin into the boiling water until dissolved.

Add the raspberry green tea powder and stir until dissolved.

Pour in the cold water and stir well.

Pour the mixture into an ice cube tray and refrigerate until set.

Nutmeg Drops

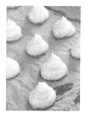

Ingredients:

6 egg whites at room temperature

2 pkgs. of Stevia sweetener

2 tbsp. fresh nutmeg, grated

Nutmeg Drops

Directions:

Preheat the oven to 400 degrees and line a baking sheet with parchment paper.

Beat the egg whites with an electric mixer until fluffy.

Sprinkle in the Stevia and continue to beat until the mixture forms stiff peaks when the beaters are lifted out of the mixture.

Drop the mixture by teaspoon full onto the prepared baking sheet.

Sprinkle the nutmeg evenly over the top of each drop.

Bake for 10 minutes or until the tops are slightly crispy and a nice golden brown.

You can use any of your favorite spices such a cinnamon, apple pie spice or pumpkin spice on these delicious treats.

Crispy Snack Chips

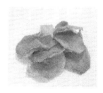

Ingredients:

2 C flat leaf kale, rinsed and dried

1 tbsp. olive oil

2 tsp. lemon juice

Directions:

Preheat the oven to 350 degrees and line a baking sheet with parchment paper.

Remove the stems from the kale and tear into bite size pieces.

In a bowl whisk together the olive oil and lemon juice.

Drizzle the mixture over the kale and toss to coat evenly.

Spread the kale over the prepared baking sheet in a single layer.

Bake the kale for 25 minutes, turning every 5 minutes, or until crispy.

Remove and allow it to cool slightly before sprinkling with a little sea salt.

Applesauce Cookies

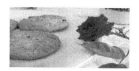

Ingredients:

1/3 C unsweetened applesauce

2 tbsp. almond paste

1 tbsp. flaxseed oil

8 packets Truvia sweetener

1 egg

½ tsp. vanilla

¾ C whole wheat flour

½ tsp. baking soda

1 tsp. cinnamon

½ tsp. salt

2 cups of quick cooking oats

½ C mixed dried fruit

½ C almonds, chopped

Applesauce Cookies

Directions:

Preheat the oven to 350 degrees and lightly spray a cookie sheet with cooking spray.

Place the applesauce, almond paste, oil and Truvia into a bowl and beat well.

Beat in the egg and vanilla.

Add the flour, baking soda and salt and stir until blended together well.

Fold in the oats, dried fruit and almonds.

Drop by teaspoonful onto the prepared cookie sheet and flatten.

Bake 15 minutes or until a nice golden brown.

Vegetable Dip

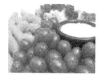

Ingredients:

2 (6 oz.) containers of plain yogurt

½ tsp. garlic powder

½ tsp. onion powder

¼ tsp. seasoned salt

Fresh vegetables

Directions:

Place the yogurt into a mixing bowl

Add the garlic powder, onion powder and salt and stir until blended in well.

Cover and refrigerate at least 30 minutes.

Serve with the assorted fresh vegetables.

Spinach Muffins

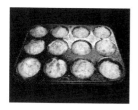

Ingredients:

1 (10 oz.) pkg. frozen spinach, thawed and squeezed dry

4 large eggs, beaten

¼ tsp. minced garlic

Spinach Muffins

Directions:

Preheat the oven to 400 degrees and line a muffin tin with paper liners.

Place the spinach into a bowl.

Add the egg and garlic.

Blend together well.

Fill each muffin cup 2/3 full.

Bake 15 minutes or until set and nicely browned.

Cool in pan 2 minutes then remove to a wire rack to cool completely.

Homemade Spice

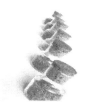

Ingredients:

1 tbsp. bay leaf, ground

2 tsp. celery salt

1 ½ tsp. dry mustard

1 tsp. pepper

1 tsp. sweet paprika

½ tsp. nutmeg

½ tsp. ginger

¼ tsp. allspice

¼ tsp. cloves, ground

¼ tsp. red pepper flakes, ground

1/8 tsp. mace, ground

1/8 tsp. cardamom, ground

Directions:

Place all the ingredients into a bowl.

Mix until well blended.

Place in a spice container and use on seafood, fish, pork or chicken.

Quick Homemade Salsa

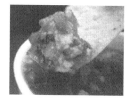

Ingredients:

1 (14.5 oz.) can diced tomatoes with jalapenos

½ onion, diced

½ tsp. cilantro

½ tsp. cumin

1 tbsp. chili powder

Directions:

Place the tomatoes with their juice into a bowl.

Add the onion and cilantro and stir to combine.

Sprinkle in the cumin and chili powder and mix together well.

Cover and refrigerate 30 minutes before serving.

CopyCat Restaurant Recipes

Uncover the Secret Recipes from Your Favorite Restaurants!

CopyCat Secret Recipes Here

http://tinyurl.com/3zznmop

Easily Prepare the Most Guarded Restaurant Recipes in Your Own Kitchen.

The same tastes and flavors for a fraction of the cost!

Copy Cat Recipes behind dishes from

Learn to cook the highly guarded secrets

» Red Lobster

» Applebee's

» Chili's

» Olive Garden

» T.G.I. Fridays

» Outback Steakhouse

» Starbucks

Made in the USA
Lexington, KY
31 October 2011